ENT

Nicholas D. Stafford MB ChB FRCS

Professor of Otolaryngology and Head and Neck Surgery, University of Hull School of Medicine, Hull, UK

Robin Youngs MD FRCS

Consultant ENT Surgeon, West Suffolk Hospital, Bury St Edmunds, UK

SECOND EDITION

CHURCHILL
LIVINGSTONE

EDINBURGH LONDON NEW YORK PHILADELPHIA SYDNEY ST LOUIS
TORONTO 1999

CHURCHILL LIVINGSTONE
An imprint of Harcourt Publishers Limited

© Longman Group UK Limited 1994
© Harcourt Publishers Limited 1999

✍ is a registered trademark of Harcourt
Publishers Limited

First published as Colour Aids—ENT 1988
Published as Colour Guide—ENT 1994
    Reprinted 1997
    Reprinted 1998
Second Colour Guide edition 1999

ISBN 0-443-06146-7

British Library Cataloguing in Publication Data
A catalogue record for this book is available from
the British Library.

Library of Congress Cataloging in Publication Data
A catalog record for this book is available from
the Library of Congress.

Medical knowledge is constantly
changing. As new information
becomes available, changes in
treatment, procedures, equipment
and the use of drugs become
necessary. The authors and the
publishers have, as far as it is
possible, taken care to ensure
that the information given in this
text is accurate and up to date.
However, readers are strongly
advised to confirm that the
information, especially with
regard to drug usage, complies
with the latest legislation and
standards of practice.

The
publisher's
policy is to use
**paper manufactured
from sustainable forests**

Printed in China.
SWTC/01

For Churchill Livingstone

Publisher: Michael Parkinson
Project Editor: James Dale
Production: Nancy Arnott
Designer: Erik Bigland

Acknowledgements

The authors are very grateful to the Department of Medical Photography at St Mary's Hospital, London, and the Departments of Medical Illustration at St Bartholomew's Hospital, London and Ipswich Hospital, for their help in obtaining material for the book. Thanks also to Mr J. Wright (Figs 32, 52, 64, and 87), Dr A. Choy (Figs 30, 35 and 41), Dr T. Lissauer (Figs 106, 140 and 156), Mr D. Archer (Figs 95 and 165), Mr N. Breach (Fig. 13), Mr D. Davies (Fig. 160), Mr J. Eyre (Fig. 116), Dr A. Forge (Fig. 54), Dr J. M. Henk (Fig. 120) and Mr P. Rhys-Evans (Fig. 121). The authors particularly appreciate the generosity of Professor Michael Hawke in offering them the use of some of his excellent tele-otoscopic pictures (Figs 9, 15, 17, 23, 27 and 34). Finally, the authors wish to express their gratitude to the patients appearing in this book, without whose cooperation this work would not have been possible.

Hull   N.D.S
1999   R.Y.

Contents

Otoscopy

The external ear should be inspected for abnormalities which may include scars from previous middle ear surgery. The external ear canal is S-shaped and can be straightened by upward and backward traction on the pinna, giving a good view of the tympanic membrane in most cases (Fig. 1). The normal tympanic membrane has a grey, translucent appearance with the handle of the malleus visible centrally (Fig. 2). The lower part of the membrane is very thin and is known as the pars tensa. In the upper part the skin is thicker and is known as the pars flaccida.

Tuning fork tests

A 512 Hz tuning fork can be used to crudely assess hearing (Fig. 3). Using the Rinne and Weber tests, a diagnosis of conductive deafness due to middle ear disease can be distinguished from sensorineural deafness due to inner ear disease.

Audiometry

Pure tone audiometry is used to measure the threshold of hearing across a range of frequencies (Fig. 4). Impedance audiometry measures the compliance of the tympanic membrane in response to changing pressure in the ear canal. In this way middle ear pressure and the presence of middle ear fluid can be assessed.

Fig. 1 Examination of the ear with an otoscope.

Fig. 2 Normal tympanic membrane.

Fig. 3 Rinne's tuning fork test of hearing.

Fig. 4 Pure tone audiometry.

2 / Congenital ear disease

External ear

Clinical features

The pinna may be absent or rudimentary (microtia) (Fig. 5). Failure of obliteration of the first branchial cleft results in a congenital sinus usually found in front of the helix or tragus (Fig. 6) which may become a site of infection requiring its excision. Accessory auricles can occur adjacent to a normally placed pinna (Fig. 7).

Middle ear

Clinical features

Ossicular chain defects often occur in association with atresia of the external auditory canal. Treacher–Collins syndrome consists of middle and external ear malformation with abnormal facial bone development.

Management

Bone anchored hearing aids and auricular prostheses (Fig. 8) have greatly improved the treatment of these conditions. particularly in bilateral cases. With this technique prostheses are secured directly to the bones of the skull via osseo-integrated screws passing through the skin.

Inner ear

Congenital defects of the inner ear usually result in severe sensorineural deafness. These disorders may have an hereditary basis. Damage to the inner ear can also be caused by events during pregnancy and the perinatal period. These include infections, particularly maternal rubella and syphilis, haemolytic disease of the newborn and fetal anoxia during birth.

Management

In the management of congenital ear disease it is vital that deafness, if present, is detected at an early stage so that treatment is instituted allowing optimum language development during early childhood.

Fig. 5 Microtia.

Fig. 6 Preauricular sinus.

Fig. 7 Accessory auricles.

Fig. 8 Bone anchored hearing aid in place.

Foreign bodies

Clinical features

Foreign bodies are most commonly found in children, e.g. beads, cotton wool buds (Fig. 9). If deeply inserted into the external ear canal, they may cause tympanic membrane perforation (Fig. 10).

Management

Removal of foreign bodies may require a general anaesthetic. Most traumatic tympanic membrane perforations heal spontaneously.

Cauliflower ear

Clinical features

Blunt trauma to the pinna may produce a subperichondrial haematoma (Fig. 11). Devoid of its blood supply, the cartilage necroses and is replaced by fibrous tissue resulting in an ugly cosmetic deformity (Fig. 12).

Management

Early drainage of the haematoma usually prevents any deformity.

Perichondritis

Perichondritis may result from open trauma, which may be surgical, involving the cartilage of the pinna or auditory meatus. Occasionally complicates a severe otitis externa.

Clinical features

Presents as a generalized red, painful and tender swelling of the pinna and oedema may also stenose the meatus. A severe facial cellulitis and necrosis of the cartilage may develop.

Management

Treatment is with antibiotics and surgical drainage of any abscess.

Fig. 9 Foreign body in the external canal.

Fig. 10 Traumatic perforation.

Fig. 11 Subperichondrial haematoma due to trauma.

Fig. 12 Cauliflower ear.

Malignant tumours

Basal cell carcinomas, squamous cell carcinomas (Fig. 13) and malignant melanomas occur on the skin of the pinna. Exposure to sunlight over a long period is a major risk factor.

Clinical features

Initially small superficial lesions progressing to deep ulceration in advanced cases. Squamous carcinomas and malignant melanomas metastasize to regional cervical lymph nodes.

Management

Treated by surgical excision, although radiotherapy is an alternative for basal and squamous carcinomas. Involvement of cartilage renders the tumour less radiosensitive.

Benign tumours

Osteomas of the external auditory meatus are most common.

Aetiology

Osteomas are associated with repeated exposure of the external auditory meatus to cold water as in swimming and diving.

Clinical features

Solitary or multiple, osteomas present as smooth swellings on the wall of the bony meatus (Fig. 14). They are often asymptomatic, but if the lumen of the meatus is occluded, retention of wax, otitis externa or hearing loss may occur.

Management

None if asymptomatic. If recurrent otitis externa occurs, osteomas may be surgically reduced.

Fig. 13 Squamous carcinoma of the pinna.

Fig. 14 Osteomas of the external auditory canal.

5 / Otitis externa

Definition	Inflammation of the skin of the external auditory meatus.
Aetiology	It is caused by either primary infection or contact sensitivity to topically applied substances such as cosmetics or antibiotics. Gram-negative organisms (e.g. *Proteus*, *Pseudomonas*) and fungi (e.g. *Aspergillus*) are often found. Precipitating factors include impacted cerumen, local trauma, middle ear discharge though a tympanic membrane perforation, swimming and skin conditions such as psoriasis and seborrhoeic dermatitis.
Clinical features	Presents as otalgia, otorrhoea and deafness. The skin of the external auditory meatus is oedematous and inflamed (Figs 15 & 16). The meatus may be occluded with discharge and in fungal infections hypae may be seen (Fig. 17). Traction on the pinna increases the otalgia, a sign not found in inflammatory conditions of the middle ear.
Management	Debris must be removed from the meatus, either by dry mopping or suction aided by the use of an operating microscope. A swab of the meatus is taken for bacteriology prior to the instillation of drops containing an antibiotic and steroid mixture. If the meatus is totally occluded, an impregnated gauze wick may be inserted. In severe cases with cellulitis spreading onto the pinna (Fig. 18) systemic antibiotics are also needed.

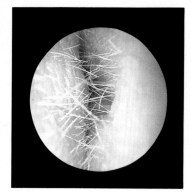

Fig. 15 Otitis externa with canal wall oedema.

Fig. 16 Bacterial otitis externa.

Fig. 17 Fungal otitis externa.

Fig. 18 Cellulitis of the pinna secondary to otitis externa.

Furunculosis of the external auditory meatus

Staphylococcal infection of hair follicles found in the lateral part of the meatus.

Clinical features

Presents as severe otalgia exacerbated by traction on the pinna, with deafness if the meatus becomes occluded. The furuncle is often visible.

Management

Most furuncles rupture spontaneously. Ribbon gauze impregnated with glycerin/ichthammol may be inserted daily into the meatus (Fig. 19). Systemic flucloxacillin and analgesics are also needed.

Malignant otitis externa

A potentially fatal *Pseudomonas* infection of the external auditory meatus. It occurs in elderly diabetics with spread to the skull base.

Clinical features

Presents as severe otalgia, otorrhoea and deafness with progression to cranial nerve palsies (VII, IX, X, XI, XII) in advanced cases.

Management

Treatment is by local surgery, usually mastoidectomy, combined with a prolonged course of specific anti-pseudomonal antibiotics. Skull base involvement and its response to treatment may be assessed by radioisotope scanning (Fig. 20).

Fig. 19 Glycerin and ichthammol wick insertion.

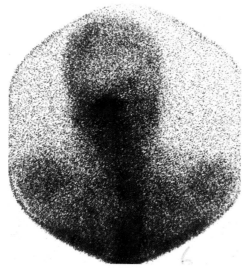

Fig. 20 Gallium scan in malignant otitis externa: increased uptake at petrous apex.

Bullous myringitis

Aetiology

An influenza virus infection of the tympanic membrane and deep external meatus, often associated with an acute otitis media.

Clinical features

Presents as otalgia, deafness and serosanguinous otorrhoea. Haemorrhagic bullae are seen on otoscopy (Fig. 21). Secondary bacterial infection can occur with purulent otorrhoea leading to otitis externa.

Management

Treat with analgesics; local and systemic antibiotics for secondary bacterial infection.

Tympanosclerosis

Aetiology

Deposits of collagen beneath the mucosa of the tympanic membrane and middle ear following otitis media or middle ear surgery, particularly grommet insertion.

Clinical features

Tympanosclerosis is mostly asymptomatic. Deposits are visible as white 'chalk patches' in the tympanic membrane (Fig. 22). Middle ear deposits may cause conductive deafness by ossicular fixation.

Management

None if asymptomatic. Ossiculoplasty may be required for conductive deafness.

Fig. 21 Bullous myringitis.

Fig. 22 Tympanosclerosis of the tympanic membrane.

7 / Middle ear effusions

Aetiology

Middle ear effusion is often associated with eustachian tube obstruction, either acute during upper respiratory infections or chronic as in childhood adenoid hypertrophy. In adults middle ear effusions may result from eustachian tube obstruction by a nasopharyngeal neoplasm. Changes in atmospheric pressure occurring during flight or diving may also result in effusions: otitic barotrauma.

Incidence

Middle ear effusion is a common paediatric problem, particularly in the 4–7 age group.

Clinical features

On otoscopy the tympanic membrane is dull with a loss of light reflex (Fig. 23). Small vessels are often seen radiating from the handle of the malleus and occasionally a fluid level is seen (Fig. 24). Deafness in children may lead to poor language development and educational performance. Diagnosis may be confirmed by impedance audiometry in which the compliance of the tympanic membrane is measured in response to pressure changes in the external auditory meatus.

Management

Medical treatment: consists of the use of topical and systemic decongestants.

Surgical treatment: consists of myringotomy and insertion of a ventilation tube into the affected tympanic membrane (Figs 25 & 26). Children may also require an adenoidectomy whilst in adults a nasopharyngeal tumour must be excluded.

Fig. 23 'Glue' ear.

Fig. 24 Serous middle ear effusion with fluid level.

Fig. 25 Grommet in situ.

Fig. 26 Types of ventilation tubes: Goode T tube, Shah and Sheppard grommets (top to bottom).

Acute otitis media

Aetiology

Acute infection of the middle ear cleft, common in young children. This usually occurs as part of an upper respiratory tract infection with *Haemophilus influenzae* and *Pneumococcus* being the most common pathogens.

Clinical features

Presents as severe otalgia and deafness. The tympanic membrane is red and bulging (Fig. 27). Rupture may occur leading to purulent otorrhoea.

Management

Treat with oral antibiotic therapy (amoxycillin, cotrimoxazole or erythromycin) and adequate analgesia.

Acute mastoiditis

Aetiology

Acute mastoiditis may complicate acute otitis media. Infection of the mastoid air cell system occurs.

Clinical features

Presents as worsening of otalgia with tenderness over the mastoid antrum. The external meatus may be narrowed by oedema of the posterior–superior wall. In advanced cases a subperiosteal abscess may push the ear forward (Fig. 28). Diagnosis is confirmed by opacity of the mastoid cells on CT scan (Fig. 29).

Management

Initially high dose parenteral antibiotic therapy is required, although in cases which fail to respond to antibiotics, or in which a subperiosteal abscess has formed, surgical drainage via a cortical mastoidectomy is required.

Fig. 27 Acute otitis media.

Fig. 28 Postauricular swelling and redness in acute mastoiditis.

Fig. 29 CT scan showing mastoid opacity in mastoiditis.

Chronic otitis media

Aetiology

Chronic inflammation of the middle ear cleft is usually associated with a perforation of the tympanic membrane. Perforations usually result from previous episodes of acute otitis media when the membrane fails to heal following rupture, but can be due to direct or indirect trauma. In children, perforations can persist following extrusion of ventilation tubes from the tympanic membrane. Organisms can reach the middle ear from the eustachian tube or from the external meatus. Chronic middle ear infection is also associated with ossicular damage with the incudostapedial joint being the most commonly affected linkage.

Clinical features

A *central perforation* in the pars tensa part of the membrane (Figs 30 & 31) is associated with recurrent otorrhoea and conductive deafness. This type of perforation is regarded as 'safe' as neurological complications are rare. An *attic* or *marginal perforation* (Fig. 32) can be associated with the development of a cholesteatoma and is regarded as 'unsafe'.

Management

Cases of central perforation should be kept dry. If recurrent otorrhoea occurs, ear drops containing a mixture of steroid and antibiotic are used and attention should be paid to possible sources of infection in the nasopharynx, nose and paranasal sinuses. A dry perforation can be repaired by myringoplasty. Traumatic central perforations usually heal spontaneously.

Fig. 30 Dry posterior central perforation.

Fig. 31 Subtotal perforation.

Fig. 32 Dry attic perforation.

A ball of keratinizing stratified squamous epithelium in the middle ear cleft or mastoid which enlarges and can destroy or erode local structures. It is a feature of the 'unsafe' type of chronic middle ear disease.

Aetiology

The most widely accepted theory of its development is the immigration–retraction pocket theory: in response to eustachian tube obstruction and negative middle ear pressure an inward retraction of the tympanic membrane occurs, usually in the attic region. Desquamated epithelium normally shed from the membrane into the meatus collects in the pocket, the continued enlargement of which results in the formation of a cholesteatoma sac. Congenital cholesteatoma is very rare (Fig. 33) and results from congenital squamous cell rests within the temporal bone.

Clinical features

Presents as progressive conductive hearing loss with purulent, and often offensive, otorrhoea. Pain or vertigo due to bony erosion may also occur. Otoscopy reveals a retraction pocket or perforation in the attic or posterior marginal region of the tympanic membrane (Fig. 34) with flaky white debris visible in the defect. Nystagmus and other evidence of neurological involvement should be sought.

Management

Radical mastoidectomy involves removal of the cholesteatoma, middle ear structures and bone of the bony external meatus, producing a smooth exteriorized mastoid cavity accessible for inspection. The operation may be modified in order to conserve hearing by retaining part of the ossicular chain and tympanic membrane (Fig. 35).

Fig. 33 Congenital cholesteatoma behind an intact tympanic membrane.

Fig. 34 Attic perforation with cholesteatoma.

Fig. 35 Healed right modified radical mastoidectomy cavity.

Extracranial

Facial nerve paralysis

Aetiology

Pressure by cholesteatoma on the facial nerve in the middle ear or mastoid.

Clinical features

Presents as partial or complete lower motor neurone facial paralysis (Fig. 36) with evidence of chronic middle ear disease on otoscopy.

Management

Treatment is by immediate surgical decompression of the facial nerve via a mastoidectomy operation.

Suppurative labyrinthitis

Aetiology

Follows erosion of the bony labyrinth most commonly over the lateral semicircular canal. In the early stages compression of the air in the external meatus causes vertigo from mechanical stimulation of the labyrinth (Fistula test). Later purulent infection in the inner ear causes severe vertigo and sensorineural deafness.

Management

Treatment is by intravenous antibiotics and eradication of cholesteatoma via mastoidectomy.

Gradenigos syndrome

Otorrhoea is associated with pain behind the eye and diplopia, caused by fifth and sixth nerve irritation resulting from air cell infection at the petrous apex (Fig. 37).

Fig. 36 Complete lower motor neurone facial palsy.

Fig. 37 Gradenigos syndrome: patient looking to right.

Intracranial

Intracranial spread of organisms may occur via the middle ear by thrombophlebitis or by penetration of the dura of the middle or posterior cranial fossae.

Meningitis

Clinical features

Presents as headache, neck stiffness and photophobia. Lumbar puncture confirms the diagnosis. *Pneumococcus* and *Haemophilus influenzae* are common pathogens.

Management

Treatment is by intravenous antibiotics followed by mastoidectomy once the meningitis has resolved.

Venous sinus thrombosis

Follows spread of middle ear and mastoid infection through the bone over the sigmoid sinus.

Clinical features

Presents as headache, pyrexia and rigors. Extension of thrombus to the superior sagittal sinus leads to CSF outflow obstruction: otitic hydrocephalus.

Management

Treatment is by intravenous antibiotics and mastoidectomy, during which infected thrombus may need to be removed from the sinus lumen (Fig. 38).

Intracranial abscess

Extradural, subdural and cerebral abscesses occur. Infection spreads into the middle and posterior cranial fossae leading to temporal lobe and cerebellar abscesses respectively. Diagnosis is by CT scan (Figs 39 & 40) and treatment by neurosurgical drainage.

Fig. 38 Lateral sinus thrombosis (MRI).

Fig. 39 CT scan showing air in the subdural space in a subdural abscess.

Fig. 40 Otogenic cerebellar abscess on CT scan.

11 / Otosclerosis

A disease primarily of the bone of the otic capsule which causes a conductive hearing loss, usually because of stapes fixation. A sensorineural deafness may occur in later stages.

Incidence

The disease is usually bilateral and presents between the ages of 15 and 45 years. Tinnitus is common and 25% of patients have positional vertigo. 70% have a family history of otosclerosis.

Clinical features

Examination of the tympanic membrane is usually normal, the pink drum (Schwartze sign) being rare and indicative of active disease (Fig. 41). In the early stages the audiogram shows a pure conductive loss, frequently with a Cahart's notch at 2000 Hz (Fig. 42).

Management

An air conduction hearing aid is frequently very successful for the patient. In the stapedectomy operation the stapes arch is replaced by a piston, usually made of Teflon (Fig. 43). Stapedectomy will produce excellent improvement in hearing level in the majority of cases, although profound deafness and vertigo are occasional complications.

A rare variant is seen in association with osteogenesis imperfecta (van der Hoeve syndrome), these patients being recognized by their blue sclera. Stapedectomy is less successful in these cases.

Fig. 41 Schwartze sign: flamingo pink flush behind tympanic membrane.

Fig. 42 Pure tone audiogram with bilateral Cahart's notches.

Fig. 43 Teflon stapes prosthesis.

Myringoplasty

Central perforations may be repaired when accompanied by deafness or recurrent middle ear infections or when an intact tympanic membrane is required for swimming or as a condition of employment. Fascia overlying the temporalis muscle is usually used (Fig. 44) and may be placed medial (underlay) or lateral (onlay) to the perforation.

Ossiculoplasty

Performed for conductive deafness where the ossicular chain has been interrupted by chronic infection, trauma or congenital deformity. Replacement ossicles may be constructed from natural or synthetic materials. Bone is the favoured material; where possible the patient's own incus remnant is remodelled and transposed.

Eradication of mastoid disease: mastoidectomy

Performed for acute mastoiditis failing to respond to high dose antibiotics, otorrhoea due to chronic mastoid infection, and middle ear and mastoid cholesteatoma.

Cortical mastoidectomy: involves exenterating the mastoid air cell system without interfering with the external meatus, ossicles or tympanic membrane (Fig. 45).

Radical and modified radical mastoidectomy: for cholesteatoma involve removal of the posterior meatal wall creating a large cavity accessible for cleaning (Fig. 46).

Fig. 44 Harvesting a temporalis fascia graft.

Fig. 45 Cortical mastoidectomy (cadaver dissection).

Fig. 46 Radical mastoidectomy (cadaver dissection).

Disruption of the lower motor neurone facial nerve can occur at any point between its brainstem nucleus and the facial musculature.

Bell's (idiopathic) palsy

Clinical features

Most common palsy with no identifiable cause although a viral or vascular aetiology postulated. Palsy may be partial or complete.

Management

Total recovery occurs in 90% of cases. Treatment with steroids or surgical decompression controversial.

Ramsay Hunt syndrome

Clinical features

Herpes zoster involvement of the facial nerve with herpetic vesicles on the tympanic membrane (Fig. 47), pinna (Fig. 48) or palate. May present with severe otalgia alone. Auditory and trigeminal nerves may be affected.

Management

Recovers fully in about 60% of cases. If given early, the antiviral agent aciclovir may enhance recovery. The value of steroids or surgical decompression of the nerve remains unproven.

Temporal bone fracture

Clinical features

Longitudinal fractures (80%) are associated with a facial palsy in 20% of cases and a conductive deafness. Transverse fractures (20%) are associated with a facial palsy in 50% of cases and a sensorineural deafness. Diagnosis is confirmed by CT scan (Fig. 49).

Management

Exploration of the nerve may be indicated in cases of immediate, complete paralysis but is likely to be followed by deafness.

Fig. 47 Herpetic vesicles on the tympanic membrane.

Fig. 48 Herpetic vesicles on the pinna.

Fig. 49 Temporal bone fracture.

Otogenic vertigo is a hallucination or a false sensation of movement. Disease affecting the vestibular apparatus may produce rotatory vertigo accompanied by horizontal nystagmus.

Testing

Caloric testing (Fig. 50).   Involves stimulating the vestibular apparatus by irrigating the external meatus with water at varying temperatures; the duration of induced nystagmus is recorded allowing comparison between the two sides.

Positional testing (Fig. 51).   Vertigo provoked by head movements (positional vertigo) may be a feature of inner ear disease, cervical spondylosis or disease affecting central vestibular pathways in the brainstem.

Ménière's disease

Aetiology

Unknown; may be due to imbalance between production and absorption of inner ear endolymph or disturbance of inner ear immunity.

Clinical features

Episodic rotatory vertigo, tinnitus and sensorineural deafness may be present. Unilateral in early stages.

Management

Treat with vestibular sedatives for acute attacks. Surgical treatment may be conservative (endolymphatic sac surgery) or destructive (labyrinthectomy or vestibular nerve section).

Sudden unilateral vestibular failure

Aetiology

Unknown aetiology. Viral infection, ischaemia and inner ear membrane rupture have been postulated.

Clinical features

Presents with sudden onset of vertigo. Recovery takes place by central compensation.

Management

Vestibular sedatives are useful in the acute phase.

Other causes of vertigo are syphilis, suppurative labyrinthitis, temporal fractures and ototoxic drugs.

Fig. 50 Caloric testing.

Fig. 51 Positional testing.

Sensorineural hearing loss results from disease in the cochlea or its central neuronal connections. The disease can be congenital (Fig. 52) or acquired.

Congenital

Aetiology

Aplasias. Partial or complete failure of inner ear development, e.g. Schiebe anomaly.

Abiotrophies. Inner ear anatomically developed but neural pathways degenerate prematurely, e.g. Pendred, Hurler and Alport syndromes.

Intrauterine/perinatal damage. Includes hypoxia, kernicterus, rubella, cytomegalovirus, syphilis, thalidomide.

Acquired

Aetiology

- Presbyacusis: the most common cause
- Noise-induced hearing loss
- Ménière's disease
- Acoustic neuroma (Fig. 53)
- Trauma, e.g. head injury, middle ear surgery
- Sudden (idiopathic) sensorineural hearing loss
- Drug-induced hearing loss, e.g. gentamicin (Fig. 54)
- Syphilis/yaws

Management

The management of any sensorineural hearing loss involves rehabilitation, once any treatable cause has been excluded. Special schooling may be necessary for the severely deaf child.

Fig. 52 White forelock in Waardenburg syndrome.

Fig. 53 Posterior fossa MRI scan showing an acoustic neuroma.

Fig. 54 Scanning electron micrograph of gentamicin-damaged cochlear hair cells.

Early diagnosis of deafness is the key to successful auditory rehabilitation, particularly in children with congenital deafness. With early intensive auditory training most children will develop the ability to communicate orally. Lip reading is an adjunct to oral communication. Manual communication, as in sign language, may be applicable for severely deaf people.

Hearing aids

Hearing aids amplify incoming sound and in some cases modify the frequency response and maximum intensity. The postaural aid (Fig. 55) is most widely used, while the body-worn aid is a bulkier but more powerful alternative. To enable parents to communicate with deaf children the 'phonic aid' (Fig. 56) has been developed in which sound is transmitted electronically over short distances.

Cochlear implants

Direct electrical stimulation of the cochlear portion of the inner ear in response to incoming sound waves has been investigated in the development of cochlear implants. Electrodes are either placed on the surface of the cochlea (extracochlear) or inserted into the lumen of the cochlea (intracochlear) (Fig. 57).

The use of cochlear implantation is established in patients with severe sensorineural deafness (e.g. post-meningitis). It is currently being evaluated in children with congenital deafness.

Fig. 55 Postaural hearing aid.

Fig. 56 Phonic aids.

Fig. 57 X-ray showing cochlear implant in situ.

Nasal obstruction, rhinorrhoea, epistaxis or facial pain may indicate intranasal or paranasal sinus disease. Clinical assessment begins with observation. Is the patient an obligatory mouth breather? Look for an obvious external nasal deformity. The nasal airway is then assessed. In children, this is undertaken using a chrome tongue depressor held just below the nose whilst the child breathes (Fig. 58). Misting of the chrome indicates a patent airway. In adults the examiner's thumb is used to close one airway at a time, being careful not to apply any lateral pressure which could occlude both sides simultaneously.

The two nasal cavities are then examined in turn using a Thudicums nasal speculum. The anterior nasal septum is assessed along with evaluation of the lateral nasal walls (Fig. 59). Only the inferior and middle turbinates can be seen by anterior rhinoscopy. The nasal mucosa is also evaluated for evidence of rhinitis.

Finally, the nasopharynx is examined. A tongue depressor is used to allow mirror examination of the nasopharynx and eustachian tube orifices. Alternatively, fibreoptic endoscopy can be employed.

Depending on the suspected pathology, the ears, larynx and neck should also be assessed.

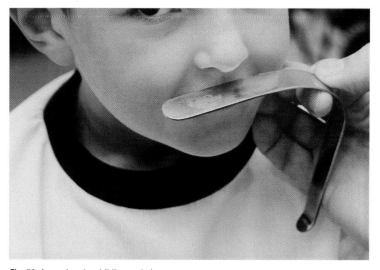

Fig. 58 Assessing the child's nasal airway.

Fig. 59 Examining the nasal cavities.

Rhinophyma

Clinical features

Red nodular masses centred around the nasal tip in association with acne rosacea (Fig. 60), usually seen in elderly men.

Management

If unsightly, treat by dermabrasion or surgical shaving.

Lupus vulgaris

Aetiology

Inoculation of the bacterium *Mycobacterium tuberculosis*, possibly through nose picking.

Clinical features

Red/brown patches or nodules on the nasal or facial skin. Perforation of the cartilaginous nasal septum can occur, with scarring in long standing cases (Fig. 61).

Management

Treatment is by antituberculous chemotherapy.

Lupus pernio

Clinical features

Skin lesions other than erythema nodosum occur in 20% of patients with sarcoidosis. Lupus pernio (Fig. 62) is common and is frequently associated with bone cysts and chest disease.

Management

Treat the underlying disease.

Malignant tumours

Clinical features

Basal or squamous cell carcinomas (Fig. 63) present as warty or ulcerating lesions, rarely with lymphadenopathy. Melanomas are more rare.

Management

Excision biopsy when possible; radiotherapy for larger tumours not involving bone.

Fig. 60 Rhinophyma.

Fig. 61 Lupus vulgaris.

Fig. 62 Lupus pernio.

Fig. 63 Squamous carcinoma.

Aetiology

Most cases of epistaxis are idiopathic, although bleeding can also result from a number of specific conditions.

Local conditions: include nasal trauma, nasal and paranasal sinus tumours and nasal septal perforations.

General conditions: include systemic bleeding diatheses such as leukaemia, anticoagulant therapy and thrombocytopenia, and systemic vascular disorders. In hereditary haemorrhagic telangiectasia (Rendu–Osler–Weber syndrome, Fig. 64), epistaxis is a prominent feature and usually arises from abnormal vessels on the nasal septum.

Systemic hypertension, although not a cause of epistaxis, is often associated with an increased severity of bleeding.

Clinical features

In most cases of epistaxis bleeding originates from the nasal septum, particularly Little's area just behind the mucocutaneous junction where there is a rich anastomosis of vessels (Kiesselbach's plexus, Fig. 65). Bleeding from a postero-superior site in the nasal cavity can occur, especially in the elderly. Haemorrhage can present via the anterior nares or pass backwards via the nasopharynx where it is spat out or swallowed. In severe cases with profuse blood loss, hypotension and tachycardia may occur. ➡

Fig. 64 Rendu–Osler–Weber syndrome.

Fig. 65 Endoscopic view of prominent blood vessels in Little's area.

Initial measures to stop bleeding consist of exerting pressure on Little's area by pinching the nose, with the patient leaning forward and spitting any blood into a bowl (Fig. 66). If a bleeding vessel is seen, it may be coagulated with chemical or electric cautery following topical application of local anaesthetic, but this is rarely successful in the acute stage. Epistaxis not responding to pressure necessitates nasal packing either with gauze impregnated with an antiseptic such as bismuth, iodoform and paraffin paste (BIPP) (Fig. 67) or with nasal balloons. Patients requiring nasal packing also require hospitalization.

In severe cases arterial ligation may be required, the available arteries being the external carotid via the neck (Fig. 68), the internal maxillary via the maxillary antrum and the anterior ethmoidal via an inner canthal incision.

An alternative to arterial ligation in severe cases is arterial embolization performed with angiographic control by a radiologist. Intravenous resuscitation with blood or plasma substitute is necessary in cases where hypotension and tachycardia are present.

Fig. 66 Pressure and posture during epistaxis.

Fig. 67 Nasal packing.

Fig. 68 External carotid artery just prior to ligation.

Deviated nasal septum

Aetiology

This occurs following previous nasal trauma or results from asymmetric septal development possibly following birth trauma.

Clinical features

Presents as unilateral nasal obstruction (Fig. 69) and less commonly epistaxis. The inferior and middle turbinates on the side opposite the septal deflection often undergo compensatory hypertrophy.

Management

If symptoms warrant, the septum can be positioned in the midline as in the operations of septoplasty and submucosal resection.

Septal haematoma

A collection of blood beneath the mucoperichondrium and posteriorly the mucoperiosteum of the nasal septum.

Aetiology

Usually complicates nasal trauma, either accidental or iatrogenic following septal surgery. Rarely a spontaneous haematoma can occur in a bleeding diathesis.

Clinical features

Presents as nasal obstruction with widening of the septum on inspection (Fig. 70).

Management

In the acute stage, treat by incision and drainage; however, after 48 h, organization of haematoma occurs and evacuation of the clot is difficult. Antibiotics are given to prevent secondary infection.

Fig. 69 Deviated nasal septum.

Fig. 70 Septal haematoma.

Septal abscess

Aetiology

Septal abscesses usually result from secondary infection of a septal haematoma.

Clinical features

Manifests by the development of severe pain, nasal swelling and pyrexia following a septal haematoma. Cartilage necrosis often complicates septal haematoma and abscess with the production of a saddle-nose deformity (Fig. 71).

Management

Treatment is by incision and drainage with appropriate antibiotic therapy.

Septal perforation

Aetiology

Traumatic: after septal surgery, nose picking, cocaine sniffing and pressure from foreign bodies and nasal polyps.

Infective: due to syphilis and tuberculosis.

Chronic inflammatory. Wegener's granulomatosis is a non-neoplastic upper airways granuloma associated with focal lung and kidney lesions. (Lethal) midline granuloma is thought to be an atypical lymphoma occurring in the midline of the face.

Clinical features

Asymptomatic, or nasal crusting and epistaxis are characteristic of septal perforation (Fig. 72).

Management

Treatment is by removal of crusts, nasal douches and treatment of underlying systemic conditions.

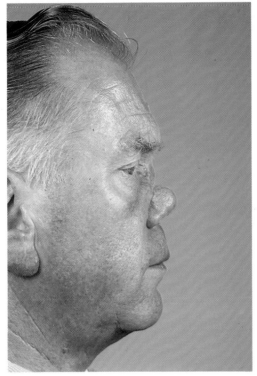

Fig. 71 Saddle-nose deformity following septal abscess.

Fig. 72 Septal perforation.

Allergic rhinitis

Aetiology

Hypersensitivity to inhaled or ingested allergens causes nasal mucosal oedema and exudation. Allergy may be seasonal (e.g. pollens) or perennial (e.g. house dust). Allergies may be demonstrated by skin tests (Fig. 73).

Clinical features

Presents as nasal obstruction, sneezing and rhinorrhoea with mucosal oedema on examination (Fig. 74).

Management

Treat with steroid nasal spray and oral antihistamines. Avoid any known allergens.

Non-allergic rhinitis

Clincial features

Presents as chronic nasal obstruction and rhinorrhoea with no demonstrable allergy.

Management

If medical treatment in the form of antihistamines or steroid sprays fails to produce relief, nasal obstruction may be helped by surgical reduction or diathermy of the inferior turbinates.

Long term use of sympathomimetic vasoconstrictor nasal sprays can result in chronic nasal congestion as a rebound effect: rhinitis medicamentosa.

Atrophic rhinitis

Aetiology

A disease of unknown aetiology, occurring mainly in developing countries. It can occur following radical turbinectomy operations or radiotherapy to the nasal cavity.

Clinical features

Nasal crusting, anosmia and fetor are present. Paradoxically, although the nasal cavity is widely patent, the sensation of nasal obstruction is common.

Management

Treatment is by removal of crusts and nasal douches.

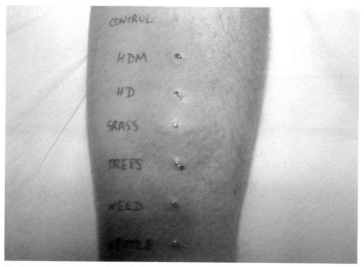

Fig. 73 Positive skin tests in allergic rhinitis.

Fig. 74 Inferior turbinate hypertrophy.

22 / Simple nasal polyps

Aetiology

Simple nasal polyps are pedunculated areas of oedematous mucosa occurring in the nasal cavity and paranasal sinuses. Their aetiology is unknown although chronic sinus infection and mucosal allergy have been suggested. Most polyps arise from the ethmoid sinuses with the maxillary antrum being a less common source.

Nasal polyps can be associated with asthma and aspirin sensitivity (aspirin triad). In children, nasal polyps may be a manifestation of cystic fibrosis.

Clinical features

Presents as progressive nasal obstruction and rhinorrhoea. On inspection of the nasal cavity, polyps are seen as pale grey smooth swellings which can fill the nasal cavity (Fig. 75). Most cases are bilateral but in unilateral cases a neoplasm must be excluded by biopsy. An antrochoanal polyp passes from the maxillary sinus via its ostium posteriorly into the nasal cavity to occupy the posterior choana where it can be seen on posterior rhinoscopy (Fig. 76) and its presence confirmed by lateral radiography.

Management

Medical treatment: topical steroid drops or spray administered correctly can cause considerable diminution in polyp size.

Surgical treatment: intranasal polypectomy (Fig. 77) may have to be repeated as recurrence after polyp removal is common. In severe cases ethmoidectomy may be required.

Fig. 75 Simple nasal polyps.

Fig. 76 Antrochoanal polyp behind soft palate.

Fig. 77 Operative specimens from one patient.

Aetiology	Stasis and acute infection of sinus secretions may result from any pathological or anatomical abnormality obstructing free sinus drainage. The common cold is the most frequent cause. Acute maxillary sinusitis can also result from apical infection of an upper tooth root. The causative organism is usually *Pneumococcus*, *Streptococcus viridans* or *Haemophilus influenzae*.
Complications	Left untreated, acute sinusitis can rarely lead to orbital cellulitis, cavernous sinus thrombosis or intracranial abscess formation (Fig. 78). Chronic sinusitis is a far more common sequela.

Maxillary sinusitis

Clinical features	Most common type overall. Facial or dental pain may occur, as may referred otalgia. Nasal obstruction and purulent rhinorrhoea are also frequent. Local tenderness may be the only physical sign. An occipitomental X-ray usually shows a fluid level on one or both sides (Fig. 79), but this investigation is increasingly being replaced by CT scanning (Fig. 80).
Management	Treat with antibiotics and topical nasal decongestants. An antral washout (Fig. 81) through the inferior meatus may be necessary if resolution with antibiotics does not occur, but this form of treatment is decreasing in popularity with the advent of endoscopic management of sinusitis.

Fig. 78 Anterior fossa extradural abscess (upper scan) secondary to frontal sinusitis (lower scan).

Fig. 79 Bilateral antral fluid levels.

Fig. 80 CT scan of maxillary sinusitis.

Fig. 81 Antral washout.

Ethmoiditis

Incidence

Most common in young children who have poorly developed maxillary sinuses.

Clinical features

Usually presents as persistent headache and orbital cellulitis (Fig. 82) following a cold. Untreated, an orbital abscess and blindness may occur.

Management

Treatment requires hospital admission. Antibiotics are given and the maxillary sinuses washed out if also infected. Rarely, an external ethmoidectomy may be necessary. A CT scan should be performed if there is any question of an orbital abscess.

Frontal sinusitis

Potentially the most serious acute sinusitis. The long course of the frontonasal duct makes it particularly prone to obstruction by mucosal oedema.

Clinical features

Presents as frontal headache after an upper respiratory tract infection. Local tenderness is common, but may be the only sign. An occipito-frontal X-ray usually shows a fluid level or complete opacification in one or both sinuses.

Management

Treatment is with antibiotics, but sinus trephine and insertion of drainage tubes (Fig. 83) is undertaken if rapid resolution does not occur.

Sphenoiditis

Clinical features

This rare form of sinusitis may present as a deep central, retro-orbital or vertex headache. Diagnosis is confirmed by a lateral X-ray or CT scan (Fig. 84). Sinus drainage may be necessary if there is not a quick response to antibiotic therapy.

Fig. 82 Acute ethmoiditis with orbital cellulitis.

Fig. 83 Surgical drainage of acute frontal sinusitis.

Fig. 84 Sphenoid sinus mucocele on CT scan.

Frontal sinusitis

Clinical features

Presents as a persistent frontal headache or, if a mucocele develops, a unilateral proptosis (Fig. 85). A pyocele may result from secondary infection of a mucocele. X-rays show an opaque sinus often with hazy, indistinct edges. A CT scan will show a soft tissue mass filling the sinus (Fig. 86).

Management

Treatment is by a fronto-ethmoidectomy, leaving a polythene tube in situ for 3 months in order to re-establish a good frontonasal duct. Further problems merit frontal sinus obliteration via an osteoplastic flap approach.

Maxillary sinusitis

Aetiology

Disease is commonly bilateral unless there is an underlying septal deviation, unilateral polyp or history of maxillary trauma. A past history of dental treatment may be relevant.

Clinical features

Usually presents with chronic facial pain or upper jaw toothache. Other presentations include a purulent postnasal drip, chronic laryngitis or otitis media. Examination is often normal but paranasal sinus X-rays usually demonstrate antral disease, in the form of mucosal thickening, a persistent fluid level or total opacification.

Management

Treatment involves the creation of intranasal antrostomies to drain the antra. If symptoms persist, endoscopic sinus surgery or a Caldwell–Luc approach can be used to remove the diseased antral mucosa (Fig. 87).

Fig. 85 Unilateral proptosis due to a mucocele.

Fig. 86 Unilateral chronic frontal sinusitis.

Fig. 87 Caldwell–Luc approach to the maxillary antrum.

The widespread availability of endoscopes and high quality radiology has led to a reappraisal of many of the established methods of treatment for chronic sinusitis. Most sinus infections are rhinogenic, spreading from the nose into the sinuses. Both the frontal and maxillary sinuses are drained and ventilated through the narrow clefts of the anterior ethmoid cells, close to the middle nasal turbinate. It is this small area which is critical in the development of chronic sinusitis.

Diagnostic evaluation

Patients with a history suggestive of chronic sinusitis are evaluated by rigid endoscopy under local anaesthetic. The middle meatus is particularly important (Fig. 88), and is inspected for evidence of polyps, purulent secretion (Fig. 89) or anatomical abnormality which may impede sinus ventilation.

Where endoscopic surgery is necessary a CT scan in the coronal plane is obtained to show the underlying sinus anatomy (Fig. 90), the extent of chronic sinus disease (Fig. 91), and its relationship to adjacent structures such as the orbital contents and anterior cranial fossa.

Endoscopic surgery

When chronic sinusitis persists despite adequate medical treatment, patients may undergo endoscopic surgery. These operations remove diseased sinus mucosa and improve ventilation in the middle meatus area. Usually anterior ethmoidectomy is performed, but in more extensive disease access to the posterior ethmoidal and sphenoidal sinuses is possible.

Fig. 88 Normal middle meatus.

Fig. 89 Pus in the middle meatus.

Fig. 90 Normal coronal CT scan.

Fig. 91 CT scan with ethmoidal disease.

Lymphoid tissue found at the junction of the roof and posterior wall of the nasopharynx, thought to be involved in the development of humoral immunity as a component of the 'gut associated lymphoid tissue' (GALT). Adenoid tissue is present at birth and during childhood, beginning to atrophy before puberty.

Clinical features

Adenoidal hypertrophy (Fig. 92) disturbs nasopharyngeal airflow and eustachian tube function and can also act as a focus of infection for adjacent sites. Common clinical features are nasal obstruction and discharge, deafness due to middle ear effusion and otalgia due to recurrent otitis media. Gross adenoidal enlargement often associated with tonsillar hypertrophy can cause sleep apnoea syndrome in which apnoeic episodes during sleep are associated with daytime somnolence and in severe cases pulmonary hypertension and cor pulmonale. Clinical suspicion of enlarged adenoids can be confirmed by lateral radiography (Fig. 93).

Management

Surgical removal (adenoidectomy) can be undertaken if enlarged adenoids are causing sleep apnoea, nasal obstruction or are a contributing factor to persistent middle ear effusions or recurrent otitis media.

Fig. 92 Operative specimen of adenoids.

Fig. 93 Adenoidal hypertrophy (arrowed).

Nasal fractures

Clinical features

This common fracture can produce an external deformity (Fig. 94) which may be palpable, and internal disruption, e.g. septal haematoma or septal deviation. Ethmoid involvement may produce CSF rhinorrhoea.

Management

Reduce any external bony deviation under general or local anaesthesia. A septal deviation may require a submucosal resection at a later date.

Zygomatic (malar) fractures

Clinical features

Usually tripartite (Fig. 95), the cheek contour is flattened and trismus is common. Orbital movements may be limited if the orbital floor is involved.

Management

Elevation of the zygoma (via a Gillies approach) may need to be supplemented by internal wiring and antral packing, through a Caldwell–Luc approach.

Maxillary (Le Fort) fractures

There are three types of maxillary or Le Fort fracture (Fig. 96):
- Type I
- Type II
- Type III.

Clinical features

Airways obstruction by the mobile bone fragment is a serious threat. Malocclusion is common.

Management

Treatment involves fixing the mobile portion using arch bars and, frequently, bilateral suspension wiring from the frontal or parietal bones.

Fig. 94 Fractured nasal bones.

Fig. 95 Zygomatic fracture after open reduction.

Fig. 96 Types of Le Fort maxillary fractures.

Angiofibroma

Incidence

A benign vascular tumour occurring in males under the age of 25 years.

Clinical features

Nasal obstruction, epistaxis and deafness due to middle ear effusion are common characteristics.

Management

Treatment is by surgical excision, facilitated by preoperative CT scanning (Fig. 97), arteriography and embolization (Fig. 98).

Malignant tumours

Incidence

Common in South East Asia where they account for 20% of all malignant tumours.

Clinical features

Presents as nasal obstruction, epistaxis and deafness. Metastasis to cervical nodes may occur prior to local symptoms becoming apparent. Cranial nerve palsies occur in advanced cases.

Pathology

Most are squamous carcinomas, although anaplastic carcinomas and lymphomas also occur.

Management

Radiotherapy following biopsy confirmation (Fig. 99), with surgery used only for cervical nodes not responding to irradiation.

Chordoma

A very rare locally invasive neoplasm arising from remnants of the fetal notochord found in the skull base. Presents with neurological, nasal and ophthalmic symptoms.

Fig. 97 CT scan showing an angiofibroma.

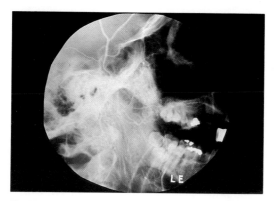

Fig. 98 Arteriogram demonstrating vascularity of angiofibroma.

Fig. 99 Endoscopic biopsy of a nasopharyngeal carcinoma.

Pathology

Benign tumours: include papillomas, adenomas, osteomas and angiomas. The inverting papilloma may undergo malignant change.

Malignant tumours: 50% of malignant tumours are found in the maxillary sinus. Squamous cell carcinoma is the most common type. Others include adenocarcinoma, adenoid cystic carcinoma, melanoma and sarcoma.

Clinical features

Benign tumours frequently present as a unilateral nasal polyp. Malignant tumours spread medially to produce nasal obstruction or epistaxis, posteriorly to give eustachian tube obstruction and cranial nerve palsies, inferiorly to disrupt the teeth (Fig. 100) or superiorly to give proptosis or epiphora. Lateral spread produces swelling of the cheek.

Management

Prior to treatment planning, histological diagnosis and radiological assessment of the extent of the tumour using CT scanning and sinus tomography are necessary (Fig. 101). Benign tumours are treated by local excision, e.g. by a Caldwell–Luc or lateral rhinotomy approach. Malignant tumours have a poor prognosis due to their late presentation and extensive spread. When curative treatment is possible a combination of radical surgery (maxillectomy) and radiotherapy is usually used. The resulting defect is filled with a dental plate and obturator (Fig. 102).

Fig. 100 Antral carcinoma involving hard palate.

Fig. 101 Extensive antral carcinoma on CT scan.

Fig. 102 Dental plate and obturator.

Nasal obstruction in children is usually noted by parents particularly when accompanied by rhinorrhoea and snoring. Adenoid hypertrophy is the most common cause of paediatric nasal obstruction; however, the following conditions should also be borne in mind.

Posterior choanal atresia

Aetiology

A congenital condition caused by persistence of the embryonic bucconasal membrane. The obstruction is at the posterior end of the nose near the edge of the hard palate.

Clinical features

In bilateral cases there is respiratory difficulty at birth aggravated by feeding and necessitating the use of an oral airway. Unilateral cases present later with unilateral nasal obstruction and rhinorrhoea. Diagnosis is made by the inability to pass a rubber catheter through the nose into the pharynx and is confirmed by CT scanning (Fig. 103).

Management

Surgical division of the atretic plate by transnasal or transpalatal route is required.

Nasal foreign body

A common occurrence in children, e.g. with beads, pieces of sponge or paper (Fig. 104).

Clinical features

Typically presents with unilateral foul blood-stained rhinorrhoea, nasal vestibulitis and fetor.

Management

A general anaesthetic is occasionally required for removal in an uncooperative child.

Fig. 103 Choanal atresia (3-D reconstruction).

Fig. 104 Foreign bodies removed from a child's nose.

Clinical features

The hallmark of laryngeal obstruction is stridor. Inspiratory stridor indicates glottic or supraglottic obstruction, expiratory stridor bronchial obstruction and two-way stridor subglottic obstruction. If stridor is accompanied by cyanosis, tachycardia and intercostal and sternal recession (Fig. 105), urgent measures are needed to save life. In less severe cases a hoarse voice, feeding problems and recurrent chest infections may occur.

Congenital laryngeal obstruction

Aetiology

Congenital anomalies include laryngeal cysts, webs, stenosis, vascular rings and vocal cord paralysis. Laryngomalacia is a condition caused by abnormal flaccidity of the larynx allowing the supraglottic structures to be drawn into the airway on inspiration; the condition resolves with age.

Management

All cases of congenital stridor should undergo direct laryngoscopy.

Acquired laryngeal obstruction

Aetiology

Acute epiglottitis: due to *Haemophilus influenzae*. It causes rapidly progressive airway obstruction (Fig. 106).

Acute laryngotracheobronchitis (croup): due to para-influenzae virus or respiratory syncitial virus. It produces oedema, exudates and crusting of the larynx, trachea and bronchi.

Subglottic stenosis: may follow infant tracheostomy or prolonged endotracheal intubation.

Management

Acute epiglottitis: treatment is with intravenous chloramphenicol. Endotracheal intubation or an emergency tracheostomy may be necessary.

Acute laryngotracheobronchitis: endotracheal intubation is rarely required.

Fig. 105 Sternal recession in a child with upper airways obstruction.

Fig. 106 Epiglottic swelling in acute epiglottitis.

Incidence	A very common disease particularly affecting children between the ages of 4 and 10 years.
Aetiology	Over 50% of the cases are due to a B haemolytic streptococcus, the majority of the others being of viral, staphylococcal or pneumococcal origin.
Clinical features	Sore throat, dysphagia, pain on swallowing and otalgia are associated with pyrexia and general malaise. The pharyngeal mucosa appears red and the tonsils are often enlarged and covered by discrete microabscesses or a confluent exudate (Fig. 107). The tonsils often remain chronically enlarged and inflamed (Fig. 108). Lymphadenopathy is frequent, the jugulo-digastric nodes being most commonly involved. A full blood count reveals a leucocytosis but a bacteriology swab does not always grow the pathogen concerned.
Differential diagnosis	*Infectious mononucleosis.* It may be impossible to distinguish between the two without a Paul–Bunnell test and a differential white cell count (the latter shows atypical monocytes and a lymphocytosis).
	Blood dyscrasias. Any white cell abnormality giving an impaired immune status may present as a severe pharyngitis, e.g. acute leukaemia.
	Diphtheria. Rarely seen but should always be borne in mind when there is a membranous exudate over the tonsils or when severe airways obstruction is evident. ➡

Fig. 107 Acute exudative tonsillitis.

Fig. 108 Chronically enlarged tonsils following recurrent infection.

Management	Bed rest, antibiotics and adequate hydration. Penicillin is given (orally or intravenously) unless organism sensitivities or allergy dictate otherwise. In severe cases with grossly enlarged tonsils a tracheostomy may be necessary for airways obstruction.

Recurrent episodes over a prolonged period of time are best managed by tonsillectomy (Fig. 109). Following surgery the tonsillar fossae heal over a period of 7–10 days during which time they are covered by a slough (Fig. 110) which may mimic an ulcerative pharyngitis. Infection and secondary haemorrhage from the fossae can occur during this period. |
| *Complications* | • Chronic tonsillitis
• Peritonsillar abscess (quinsy) (Fig. 111): hospitalization, antibiotics and intraoral incision and drainage are required
• Parapharyngeal abscess: requires surgical drainage through an external neck incision
• Acute otitis media
• Post-streptococcal rheumatic fever/glomerulonephritis: now rare |

Fig. 109 Dissection tonsillectomy using bipolar diathermy.

Fig. 110 Post-tonsillectomy slough overlying tonsillar fossae.

Fig. 111 Left-sided quinsy.

Acute retropharyngeal abscess

Lymphadenitis of the retropharyngeal nodes following an upper respiratory tract infection in children.

Clinical features

Presents with sore throat, pyrexia and swelling of the posterior pharyngeal wall. Lateral X-ray shows retropharyngeal swelling (Fig. 112).

Management

The abscess should be drained via the mouth with precautions taken to avoid inhalation of pus.

Chronic retropharyngeal abscess

Occurs in adults in association with tuberculous cervical spine disease.

Clinical features

Swelling is seen in the midline of the pharynx and X-rays show vertebral disease.

Management

Treatment is with antituberculous chemotherapy.

Parapharyngeal abscess

The tissue space lateral to the pharynx may become infected by spread of organisms from the tonsils or lower third molar teeth.

Clinical features

Presents with sore throat and trismus. The tonsil is pushed medially and there is neck swelling (Fig. 113).

Management

Treatment is by incision and drainage via the neck followed by appropriate antibiotic therapy.

Ludwig's angina

Clinical features

Cellulitis of the submandibular space secondary to dental disease or tonsillitis presents with swelling of the submental region (Fig. 114) and floor of the mouth.

Management

Treat with high dose antibiotics.

Fig. 112 Retropharyngeal abscess.

Fig. 113 Parapharyngeal abscess.

Fig. 114 Ludwig's angina.

Lingual thyroid

Aetiology

Tissue originating from the site of the foramen caecum invaginates and migrates down into the lower neck to form the thyroid gland. Thyroid tissue may be found at any point along this path of descent, e.g. lingual thyroid (Fig. 115) or thyroglossal cyst.

Clinical features

Usually presents as dysphagia. Haemorrhage and airway obstruction rarely occur.

Management

Once functioning thyroid tissue has been demonstrated elsewhere in the neck, the lump may be removed if it is causing significant symptoms.

Black hairy tongue

Aetiology

Caused by overgrowth and elongation of the filiform papillae of the anterior tongue in association with their black or brown discoloration (Fig. 116).

Clinical features

Asymptomatic, but for its appearance.

Management

Treatment is by mechanical brushing or scraping of the dorsum of the tongue.

Geographic tongue

Incidence

Affects 1% of the population.

Clinical features

Irregularly shaped areas of depapillation occur over the dorsum of the tongue (Fig. 117). The patches vary in size and distribution over a period of days.

Management

No treatment is required.

Fig. 115 Lingual thyroid.

Fig. 117 Geographic tongue.

Fig. 116 Black hairy tongue.

Leukoplakia

A white patch which cannot be wiped away and for which no other diagnosis is apparent (Fig. 118). Risk factors in the development of oral cavity or tongue leukoplakia include alcohol, smoking, spice and betelnut chewing, syphilis and dental trauma. About 5% of cases become malignant. Exclusion of an associated carcinoma is essential.

Tongue carcinoma

Almost all tongue carcinomas are squamous in origin. There need not be any pre-existing leukoplakia.

Clinical features

May present as an exophytic or infiltrative lump on the tongue (Fig. 119). Pain and dysphagia are common. Referred otalgia (via lingual and glossopharyngeal nerves) may also occur. At presentation most tumours are greater than 2 cm diameter and 50% have palpably involved lymph nodes.

Management

Small lesions. Radiotherapy, using external beam or interstitial implant techniques (Fig. 120), or surgery, in the form of a partial or hemiglossectomy (Fig. 121) are equally effective.

Large lesions. Treatment is with radiotherapy or surgery alone or a planned combination of the two. Both modalities produce quite severe functional disability in the oral cavity, especially regarding speech and swallowing.

Fig. 118 Leukoplakia of the tongue.

Fig. 119 Ulcerative tongue carcinoma.

Fig. 120 Interstitial implant in the tongue.

Fig. 121 Tongue after hemiglossectomy.

Benign cysts

Clinical features

Mucous retention cysts, tonsilloliths or cysts of inspissated epithelial debris may occur. They are smooth and localized to one portion of the tonsil (Fig. 122).

Management

Symptomatic cysts may be helped by tonsillectomy.

Lymphoma

Clinical features

Unilateral tonsillar swelling with an intact overlying mucosa (Fig. 123) may cause dysphagia and is suspicious of a lymphoma. The tonsil feels rubbery. Excision biopsy confirms the diagnosis.

Management

After staging the disease, treatment involves radiotherapy for localized disease, with chemotherapy being added in more advanced cases.

Carcinoma

Clinical features

Squamous carcinoma of the tonsil presents as otalgia, sore throat or dysphagia in heavy drinkers and smokers. More than 50% of cases have involved neck nodes ipsilaterally: this may be the mode of presentation. The tonsil is hard and ulcerated (Fig. 124).

Management

After full endoscopy and biopsy small primaries without nodes are best treated by radiotherapy. Surgery (which involves a block dissection of neck, partial mandibulectomy and excision of the primary) is reserved for radiation failures and large primaries.

Fig. 122 Tonsil retention cyst.

Fig. 123 Tonsil lymphoma.

Fig. 124 Carcinoma of the right tonsil.

Torus palatinus

Clinical features

Presents as a unilobular or multilobular bony protruberance in the midline of the hard palate (Fig. 125). The aetiology is unknown.

Management

The torus can be reduced by drilling if a denture needs to be worn or if the swelling interferes with eating.

Palatal tumours

Although these are usually due to inferior extension of a maxillary sinus tumour, benign or malignant neoplasms can arise from the palate itself (Fig. 126).

Clinical features

Presents with loose teeth, ill-fitting dentures and facial swelling. The most common types are the pleomorphic adenoma, adenoid cystic carcinoma and squamous carcinoma.

Management

Treatment is by surgical excision and/or radiotherapy, depending on the histological diagnosis.

Clefts of the palate and lip

Two of the most common congenital anomalies.

Clinical features

Clefts of the lip and palate can occur in isolation (Fig. 127) but they often occur together. Initial difficulties may be encountered with feeding, with abnormal facial development later. Palatal clefts are often associated with middle ear effusions owing to eustachian tube dysfunction.

Management

Plastic surgical repair of clefts with long-term orthodontic care and screening for middle ear effusions.

Fig. 125 Torus palatinus.

Fig. 126 Pleomorphic adenoma of the hard palate.

Fig. 127 Untreated cleft palate in an adult.

If symptoms of hoarseness, dysphagia, chronic sore throat or a lump in the neck continue for longer than 6 weeks, careful examination of the upper airway is mandatory. Listen to the patient's voice: is it intermittently or permanently dysphonic? The former might suggest a functional problem, the latter an organic one. A 'breathy' voice is typical of a vocal cord palsy. Also, listen for evidence of stridor. A 'hot potato' voice is indicative of supraglottic or oropharyngeal pathology.

When assessing the oral cavity and oropharynx, particular attention should be paid to mucosal ulceration or swelling. If the patient has a particularly brisk gag reflex, the palate and oropharynx should be sprayed with Xylocaine prior to attempting indirect laryngoscopy. A warmed laryngeal mirror is used to visualize the larynx while the doctor gently holds the patient's protruded tongue (Fig. 128). The patient should mouth breathe. Vocal cord movement is assessed by asking the patient to say 'Hey!' If the technique is not tolerated, then the patient's better nasal airway is locally anaesthetized and a fibre-optic scope used to examine the larynx and pharynx (Fig. 129).

Both the nose and neck should be routinely examined as part of the assessment of the upper airway.

Fig. 128 Indirect laryngoscopy.

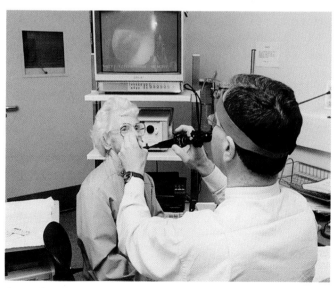

Fig. 129 Fibre-optic endoscopy.

Chronic non-specific laryngitis

Aetiology

Common. Usually associated with vocal abuse, smoking or sepsis elsewhere in the respiratory tract, e.g. chronic sinusitis.

Clinical features

Hoarseness may be accompanied by sore throat. Indirect laryngoscopy may distinguish localized forms, e.g. singer's nodules (Fig. 130), Reinke's oedema (Fig. 131) or laryngeal polyps from the generalized forms, e.g. chronic hypertrophic laryngitis (Fig. 132).

Management

Treatment involves the removal of any precipitating factors and speech therapy is important. Localized polyps or nodules may merit endoscopic removal.

Chronic specific laryngitis

Rare. Most of the granulomatous diseases can involve the larynx, e.g. tuberculosis, syphilis, sarcoidosis, scleroma or Wegener's granulomatosis.

Management

The lesions may mimic a carcinoma and a direct laryngoscopy and biopsy is mandatory. Treatment is that of the underlying systemic condition.

Leukoplakia

Usually affects the true cords (Fig. 133). The aetiology is as for chronic non-specific laryngitis. Microscopically, the findings of hyperkeratosis and dysplasia are common, although in situ or invasive carcinoma can only be excluded by an adequate biopsy.

Management

Endoscopy should be undertaken in all cases. Leukoplakia should be regarded as having the potential to undergo malignant change.

Fig. 130 Singer's nodules.

Fig. 131 Unilateral Reinke's oedema.

Fig. 132 Chronic hypertrophic laryngitis.

Fig. 133 Leukoplakia of the left true vocal cord.

Papilloma

Aetiology

Localized infection with the human papillomavirus (HPV).

Clinical features

In the child (juvenile form):   multiple lesions which may spread to the trachea and bronchi. Cases may regress at puberty.

In the adult: less common and usually a single lesion.

Both forms present with hoarseness or airway obstruction.

Management

Endoscopic removal (Fig. 134) using either suction diathermy or a CO_2 laser. Surgical seeding of lesions within the larynx or trachea is common, and removal may be necessary for frequent recurrence.

Carcinoma

Aetiology

Associated with cigarette smoking and high alcohol intake, although the latter is more important in causing piriform fossa carcinoma.

Clinical features

Usually presents as persistent hoarseness. Dysphagia, chronic cough, stridor and referred otalgia may also occur. Occasionally a supraglottic tumour may present with metastatic neck nodes. The tumour may be evident on indirect laryngoscopy but endoscopic assessment (Fig. 135) and biopsy are mandatory before deciding on the appropriate treatment. A second primary (1%) in the upper aerodigestive tract should be searched for at this time. Fine needle aspiration cytology of any suspicious neck mass should also be undertaken. A CT scan will show any spread outside the larynx, or involvement of laryngeal cartilages. ➡

Fig. 134 Endoscopic appearance of laryngeal papillomata.

Fig. 135 Early right vocal cord carcinoma.

Small (T_1 and T_2) carcinomas are best treated with primary radiotherapy, laryngectomy being reserved for post-radiation recurrences, larger (T_3 and T_4) lesions (Fig. 136) and primary tumours associated with neck nodes greater than 2 cm in diameter.

Voice rehabilitation

Following total laryngectomy the patient may be able to speak again by:
- learning oesophageal speech (swallowed air is voluntarily regurgitated through the pharynx)
- using an artificial larynx (Fig. 138) which transmits vibrations into the pharynx and oral cavity while the patient articulates
- surgical provision of a tracheo-oesophageal fistula which is fitted with a button or valve (Fig. 137). The button has a one-way flutter valve which allows airflow from the trachea into the pharynx when the tracheostome is occluded. In selected patients this enables the development of good voice.

Results

Patients require close follow-up. Recurrences can develop in the larynx, pharynx, stoma or neck. Further surgery or radiotherapy may be indicated. The expected 5-year survival for a T_1 laryngeal cancer is about 95%. This falls to about 50% for T_4 disease.

Fig. 136 Operative specimen showing extensive laryngeal carcinoma.

Fig. 137 Blom–Singer valve in situ.

Fig. 138 Patient using an 'artificial larynx'.

Oropharynx

Fish bones may lodge in the tonsil or tongue base.

Clinical features

The patient complains of pain on swallowing and points to the suprahyoid region. The bone may only be obvious on palpation: X-rays are unhelpful.

Management

Removal under direct vision.

Hypopharynx/oesophagus

A bone or food bolus usually gets lodged at one of four sites:
- one piriform fossa
- the postcricoid region (15 cm from the upper incisor)
- the level of the aortic arch (at 25 cm)
- at the oesophago-gastric junction (40 cm).

Clinical features

Dysphagia may be total, the patient spitting out saliva and pointing to the suprasternal or retrosternal region. A soft tissue lateral X-ray of the neck may delineate a bone (Fig. 139).

Management

Endoscopic removal should be undertaken as soon as possible, to avoid airway oedema, soft tissue infection or oesophageal perforation.

Bronchus

Often a peanut in a young child.

Clinical features

After an initial coughing fit there is often a latent period before respiratory distress becomes obvious. The chest X-ray may show collapse of the lung distally, if the obstruction is complete, or emphysema of the involved side if the obstruction acts as a one-way valve (Fig. 140).

Management

Bronchoscopic removal is mandatory.

Fig. 139 Chicken bone in hypopharynx.

Fig. 140 Peanut in right main bronchus, demonstrating ipsilateral emphysema.

Thyroglossal cyst

Most common midline neck cyst (Fig. 141) usually presenting in childhood.

Clinical features

Painless, unless infected, and moves on protrusion of tongue. Sinus formation may follow previous infection or incomplete excision.

Management

If a thyroid scan shows functioning tissue elsewhere, then excise with central portion of hyoid bone and tract up to foramen caecum (Sistrunk's operation).

Branchial cyst and fistula

Aetiology

Represent branchial apparatus remnants. The fistula results from persistence of the second pouch and cervical sinus.

Clinical features

Cysts usually lie deep to the anterior border of sternomastoid, presenting with a painless neck swelling or mimicking a parapharyngeal abscess if infection occurs. A complete branchial fistula has its internal opening in the region of the tonsil and an external opening anterior to sternomastoid. Diagnosis can be confirmed by needle aspiration of cyst contents.

Management

Excision, with any fistulous tract.

Cystic hygroma

A variety of lymphangioma.

Clinical features

A soft, transilluminable mass usually presenting in the parotid region in the first year of life (Fig. 142).

Management

Excision, which may have to be incomplete due to the diffuse infiltration of soft tissues by the tumour.

Fig. 141 Thyroglossal cyst.

Fig. 142 Cystic hygroma of the right parotid gland.

A tracheostomy is an artificial opening made into the trachea. It may be created after the larynx has been removed, when it is permanent, or when the larynx is still in place, when it is usually temporary (Fig. 143).

Indications

- Total laryngectomy
- Airway protection, e.g. after major head and neck surgery, neurological disease involving larynx
- Airway obstruction, e.g. epiglottitis, bilateral recurrent laryngeal nerve palsy, tumour
- Respiratory insufficiency (when endotracheal intubation required for longer than 72 h), e.g. severe chest wall injury, Guillain–Barré syndrome

Surgical technique

- Incision. Horizontal, midway between the cricoid cartilage and suprasternal notch.
- Vertical incision and separation of strap muscles.
- Transfixion and separation of thyroid isthmus.
- Creation of an opening into the trachea. In adults a window is cut out (Fig. 144). A vertical slit incision is used in children. A trap-door flap should not be used.
- Insertion of tracheostomy tube. A correctly sized cuffed synthetic tube is used for the first 24 h. This can be replaced later on by an uncuffed tube (Fig. 145). ➤

Fig. 143 Types of tracheostomy.

Fig. 144 Window cut in anterior tracheal wall.

Fig. 145 Silicone tracheostomy tubes: paediatric uncuffed and adult cuffed.

Immediate.   Pneumothorax, haemorrhage, surgical emphysema and tube displacement can all occur.

Early.   Wound infection, dysphagia and tube obstruction are all common. Tracheal erosion with innominate artery rupture, perichondritis and apnoea in hypercapnoeic bronchitics are rare.

Late.   Tracheal stenosis may result from prolonged or overinflation of the cuffed tube. Decannulation may be difficult in children. Surgical closure of a persistent tracheocutaneous fistula is rarely required after decannulation.

Stomal stenosis

Aetiology

Following laryngectomy the lower end of the trachea is brought out through the neck skin. Local wound infection, radiotherapy, and keloid formation all predispose to the later development of a stomal stenosis (Fig. 146). The other cause of stomal stenosis is recurrence of tumour (Fig. 147).

Management

Management of benign stomal stenosis is either by the permanent wearing of a stoma button or laryngectomy tube or by surgical revision of the stoma.

Fig. 146 Stomal stenosis due to scar tissue.

Fig. 147 Post-laryngectomy stomal recurrence.

Pharyngeal pouch

Aetiology

A pharyngeal pouch develops from a herniation of pharyngeal mucosa through Killian's dehiscence.

Clinical features

Dysphagia and regurgitation of food occur. Large pouches may cause aspiration pneumonia. Pooling of saliva in the hypopharynx may be noted on indirect laryngoscopy. Barium swallow confirms the diagnosis (Fig. 148).

Management

Following an endoscopy to exclude an associated carcinoma, the pouch may be excised via an external approach or the wall between the pouch and oesophagus divided endoscopically using a stapling gun (Fig. 149).

Laryngocele

Aetiology

Distension of the laryngeal saccule can produce an internal or an external laryngocele (Fig. 150).

Clinical features

Hoarseness or dysphagia may occur. External laryngoceles may produce a swelling in the neck accentuated by performing Valsalva's manoeuvre. Laryngeal tomograms taken during this manoeuvre will demonstrate the laryngocele (Fig. 151).

Management

Following endoscopy to exclude an associated carcinoma, an internal laryngocele can be 'uncapped' whilst an external laryngocele is excised through the neck.

Fig. 148 Barium swallow demonstrating a pharyngeal pouch.

Fig. 149 The use of an endoscopic stapling gun for the treatment of a pharyngeal pouch.

Fig. 150 Patient with an external laryngocele.

Fig. 151 Tomogram outlining air-filled laryngocele.

Anatomy
Formed largely by the anterior two-thirds of the tongue and by reflection of mucosa from the sides of the tongue to the gum on the mandible. In the midline the lingual frenulum separates the orifices of the left and right submandibular ducts. Under the mucosa lie the sublingual salivary glands.

Ranula

Aetiology

A cystic lesion arising from the sublingual gland. Usually presents in the floor of the mouth as a bluish, fluctuant swelling (Fig. 152). Less commonly the 'plunging ranula' can present as a lump in the neck.

Treatment

For lesions confined to the floor of the mouth, marsupialization is usually adequate, although recurrence can occur. Plunging ranulae require formal excision via an external neck approach.

Squamous carcinoma

Clinical features

An ulcer in the floor of the mouth which may be painful with referred otalgia (Fig. 153). Early spread to cervical nodes, which may be bilateral, is common.

Treatment

Excision of the tumour with plastic surgical reconstruction and adjuvant radiotherapy.

Fig. 152 Ranula of the floor of the mouth.

Fig. 153 Carcinoma of the floor of the mouth.

The superficial portion of the gland lies on the myelohyoid muscle; the deep portion extends around the posterior edge of muscle into the floor of the mouth. Wharton's duct leaves the deep part of the gland and runs forward to open into the anterior floor of the mouth, just lateral to the midline.

Swelling of the gland may be due to inflammation of tumour (Fig. 154).

Inflammatory disease

Clinical features

A tense, tender swelling usually results from a stone in the duct. This may be palpable bi-manually or evident on X-ray (Fig. 155). There are several lymph nodes in the submandibular triangle and enlargement of these may mimic disease in the gland.

Management

Treatment is with antibiotics and excision of the stone perorally. If this cannot be achieved, the whole gland may need to be removed by an external approach. Established infection may proceed to abscess formation.

Tumours

Fine needle aspiration of the mass should be performed. About 50% of tumours are benign, most commonly pleomorphic adenomas.

Management

These should be excised with the entire gland, taking care to preserve the marginal mandibular branch of the facial nerve. Malignant tumours necessitate excision of the whole gland, with a radical neck dissection in certain cases.

Fig. 154 Enlargement of the submandibular gland due to chronic infection.

Fig. 155 Floor of mouth X-ray demonstrating a stone in the submandibular gland duct.

Mumps

Clinical features

Usually seen in children, this is the most common cause of bilateral parotid gland swelling (Fig. 156). The glands are painful and tender.

Management

Treatment is supportive, the adenopathy subsiding over a period of several days.

Acute parotid abscess

Usually seen in association with poor oral hygiene, with or without dental caries.

Clinical features

The gland becomes acutely tender with obvious inflammation of the soft tissues (Fig. 157). A stone may be palpable in the duct or evident on plain X-ray.

Management

Treatment with antibiotics should be followed by drainage via a parotidectomy approach if the swelling becomes fluctuant.

Parotid gland tumours

Types

Benign: e.g. pleomorphic adenoma (Fig. 158), Warthin's tumour

Malignant: e.g. adenoid cystic, squamous cell or adenocarcinoma, lymphoma

Clinical features

Usually painless, the speed of growth reflects the likelihood of malignancy. A facial palsy indicates a malignant tumour. Fine needle aspiration of the mass may facilitate preoperative diagnosis.

Management

Superficial parotidectomy should be undertaken when indicated. Malignant tumours may require a total parotidectomy with sacrifice of the facial nerve.

Fig. 156 Mumps parotitis.

Fig. 157 Acute parotid abscess.

Fig. 158 Pleomorphic adenoma of the parotid gland.

Following excision of a tumour from the head or neck, primary closure of a resultant tissue defect with preservation of adequate function may not be feasible or cosmetically acceptable. Only by the introduction of tissue from another site can a satisfactory result be achieved. Such tissue may be used to provide lining (reconstruction of an internal mucosal defect) or cover (reconstruction of a skin defect).

Techniques

Non-vascularized free grafts.   These depend on the recipient site for their blood supply: include split skin, full thickness skin, dermis, nerve and bone grafts.

Pedicled skin.   May be random, with a non-specific blood supply, or axial, when the flap has a named arterial blood supply, e.g. deltopectoral flap (Fig. 159) and pectoralis major myocutaneous flap (Fig. 160).

Revascularized free grafts.   The artery and vein supplying the graft tissue are re-anastomosed to vessels at the recipient site. Include radial forearm flap (Fig. 161) and jejunum.

Pedicled viscera.   Stomach or colon may be used.

Several factors will determine the choice of flap/graft for the individual patient.

Myocutaneous flaps and revascularized free grafts have meant that the lining of an internal surface can be carried out as a one-stage procedure, greatly reducing hospitalization time.

Fig. 159 Neck skin replacement using a deltopectoral flap.

Fig. 160 Pectoralis major flap just prior to division of the muscles' attachments.

Fig. 161 Intra-orally placed radial free flap.

Aetiology

Often involved with lesions in the brainstem or at the skull base, e.g. with CVA, motor neurone disease, glomus tumour, meningitis and nasopharyngeal carcinoma.

Glossopharyngeal nerve

This nerve is sensory to the posterior third of the tongue (including taste) and pharyngeal mucosa. Motor to middle constrictor.

Clinical features

It is rarely paralysed alone. A unilateral palsy does not produce severe functional disability.

Vagus nerve

This nerve is sensory to the larynx and motor to the soft palate, pharynx and larynx. Also sensorimotor to the thoraco-abdominal viscera.

Aetiology

An isolated palsy of the recurrent laryngeal branch is usually either idiopathic or due to disruption of the nerve in the neck or chest, e.g. post-thyroidectomy and bronchial carcinoma (Fig. 162).

Clinical features

Variable. Palatal paralysis, hoarseness, weak cough, overspill of food and secretions and airways obstruction may all occur, although a recurrent laryngeal nerve palsy will not produce palatal paralysis.

Management

Airway incompetence due to a unilateral cord palsy may be helped by injection of Teflon into the para-cordal tissues to increase the cord's bulk or a thyroplasty could be performed (Fig. 163). Bilateral palsies may produce total airways obstruction or serious overspill. A tracheostomy will be required in either case.

Fig. 162 Bronchial carcinoma causing a left vocal cord palsy.

Fig. 163 Teflon gun for endoscopic injection of a paralysed vocal cord.

Accessory nerve

The spinal part of this nerve is motor to sternomastoid and trapezius. An isolated palsy is seen after a block dissection of neck or injudicious posterior triangle lymph node biopsy.

Clinical features

The shoulder assumes a dropped appearance (Fig. 164) and the patient is unable to shrug or abduct the shoulder to a vertical position.

Management

A resultant frozen shoulder may benefit from physiotherapy.

Hypoglossal nerve

This nerve is motor to tongue and hyoid depressors. An isolated palsy is usually iatrogenic, e.g. following laryngectomy or submandibular gland excision, or due to malignant disease in the upper neck.

Clinical features

On protrusion the tongue deviates to the paralysed side (Fig. 165). Wasting and fasciculation indicate lower motor neurone damage. Unilateral palsies are usually asymptomatic. Bilateral palsies produce severe dysarthria and swallowing difficulties.

Fig. 164 Dropped shoulder following right neck dissection (and laryngectomy).

Fig. 165 Hypoglossal nerve palsy with deviation and wasting of hemitongue.

ENT manifestations of HIV infection commonly fall into one of three groups.

Cervical lymphadenopathy

Clinical features

Common. May be persistent generalized lymphadenopathy (PGL) or secondary to pharyngitis. However, rapidly enlarging, asymmetrical (Fig. 166) or fixed nodes may herald a lymphoma, Kaposi's sarcoma or an occult squamous carcinoma.

Management

In cases where malignancy requires exclusion, fine needle or open biopsy is necessary. The treatment will then depend on the pathological diagnosis.

Kaposi's sarcoma (KS)

The skin and mucosa of the head and neck are common sites for KS in AIDS patients.

Clinical features

Lesions present as red or purple macules, plaques or nodules. Palatal involvement is most common (Fig. 167). Rarely, KS may cause airway obstruction.

Management

Treatment is multi-modal.

Oral cavity 'hairy' leukoplakia

Clinical features

Leukoplakic patches on the lateral border and ventral surface of the tongue (Fig. 168) which have a tendency to regress and recur. Possibly caused by the Epstein–Barr virus (EBV). Microscopically the keratin whorls give a hairy appearance. The lesion should be distinguished from candidiasis, also common in these patients. Rapid progression to full blown AIDS is common once 'hairy' leukoplakia has developed.

Management

Treatment is by biopsy and observation of the lesion, whose malignant potential remains unknown.

Fig. 166 Asymmetrical cervical lymphadenopathy in PGL.

Fig. 167 Kaposi's sarcoma of the hard palate.

Fig. 168 Hairy leukoplakia of the lateral border of the tongue.

Index